# Extra Views

Incidental Findings at a Community Hospital.

## Dr. Timothy A. Dunn DO

ISBN: 1481186752

ISBN 13: 9781481186759

Library of Congress Control Number: 2012923787
CreateSpace Independent Publishing Platform
North Charleston, SC

**Extra Views**
**Incidental Findings at a Community Hospital.**

*No physician, in so far as he is a physician, considers his own good in what he prescribes, but the good of his patient; for the true physician is also a ruler having the human body as a subject, and is not a mere money-maker; that has been admitted?*

Plato, The Republic

Dedicated to health care providers who chose the medical profession for the right reasons.

# Introduction

Extra Views is an autobiographical account of my experiences as a practicing radiologist. The name of the hospital in my book, Wilno General Hospital, is fictional, as are the names of all of the individuals. The events I describe occurred at two separate hospitals. In order to not complicate the story line unnecessarily, I presented my story as taking place at a single hospital. Extra Views is a composite story of my experiences. The descriptions of events and conversations are real and authentic.

Many of the challenges that health care providers face come from outside of the medical community. Political influences play a large role. For example, tort reform is largely a political issue. Physicians have been calling for tort reform for decades, to no avail. In order to placate trial lawyers, President Obama's Affordable Care Act completely ignores the issue. As a result, physicians continue to pay huge amounts of money for malpractice insurance. They also continue to practice defensive medicine. They feel compelled to order expensive tests, such as CT scans, to protect themselves from frivolous lawsuits. Efforts have been made to reduce the excessive utilization of medical technology without addressing one of the most important reasons it occurs in the first place.

There have been many attempts to replace the fee-for-service system. We saw the emergence of HMO gatekeepers, capitation, diagnostic related groups (DRG), the pay for performance program, and the infamous gag order, whereby a physician can be fired from a health care plan if he or she informs a patient of a treatment plan outside of the approved list of options. These measures had the perverse effect of financially rewarding physicians who provided less care. Nonmedical professionals, including our government and hospital administrations, often view health care as a conventional business. Their solution is to further reduce payments to providers. Medicare payments are already so low that senior citizens find it difficult to find a doctor to care for them, and reimbursements will continue to decline.

One of the great myths of health care reform is the idea that higher quality will lead to significantly lower costs. This may be true for certain specific examples. Programs that focus on smoking cessation and reducing complications in hospitalized patients fall into this category. Overall, however, higher quality requires higher costs. Preventive care involves extra expenses, in the form of screening tests, medications, and patient education. Many of my clinical colleagues have explained to me that they can provide better care, or cheaper care, but not both. This inconvenient fact runs counter to the vague and simplistic assertion that higher quality will somehow reduce costs.

Physicians are trapped between conflicting agendas. They are under pressure to utilize fewer expensive diagnostic tests and procedures, but doing so may expose them to greater medical liability. The Electronic Medical Record system (EMR) may improve efficiency, but it may be too expensive for solo practitioners. Senior citizens deserve care, but Medicare reimbursements remain low. As a result, physicians cannot accept too many of them as patients.

When these pressures are added to the considerable stresses of patient care, night call, and maintaining an office, I am not joking when I predict that increasing numbers of doctors will opt for early retirement.

Early in my career I had the pleasure of collaborating with our hospital administration in an atmosphere of mutual respect and trust. Then, in 1997, the status of health care providers was reduced to the level of blind servitude. Doctors who hesitated to join lockstep with administrative policy were labeled as troublemakers.

In my story, the culture of cost containment pervaded the hospital administration. CEO Martin Gesso, and executive vice president George Gravy (again, fictional names) claimed they were merely implementing policies made necessary by the profligate spending of the current providers. I believed that their real agenda was to enrich themselves. They wanted to run the hospital according to the pure business model, in which short term capital expenditures, such as new equipment, must be reduced, and revenues must be increased, at any cost. Administration would then take credit for being more profitable and would find the justification for their year end bonuses. In any event, that is my interpretation.

My overall opinion is that doctors are generally feeling pressures that are threatening their autonomy and economic viability, but I leave it to other physicians to decide if their experiences are similar to mine.

Extra Views is not an academic analysis of health care reform. I am a thoughtful person but I do not consider myself a health care expert. My book is a personal account of how some of the challenges described above impacted myself and some of my colleagues as we struggled to survive developments completely outside of our control. My purpose in writing my book was to educate the reader, as well as to expose certain developments, but I hope the reader also finds Extra Views entertaining.

# Chapter 1

## October 15, 1997

I was sitting near the back of the auditorium at the general medical staff meeting. The four other members of the radiology department were seated next to me, and we were getting restless. We were required by the hospital bylaws to attend these meetings, which were usually a waste of time. Tonight's meeting was no exception. The staff had already expressed several grievances, including a complaint by a stout scrub nurse that there were no XXXL scrub suits in the nurses' locker room, another that the sides of some doctors' cars had been keyed in the physicians' parking lot, and finally that some physicians were leaving dirty dishes in the doctors' dining room.

The WGH chief executive officer, Martin Gesso, began to address the general medical staff. He was joined at the front of the auditorium by the five members of the board of directors, who had never before attended a staff meeting. The board consisted of an elite group of members of the Rainbow Valley Country Club who considered themselves to be politically correct and best qualified to direct the affairs of the hospital, even though they knew nothing about the field of medicine. Their base of operation was the golf course. They were present at the staff meeting as a show of force. The word was out that there was going to be a cultural change at the hospital in the coming year.

Martin Gesso had been CEO for exactly one month. His previous job was vice president of an office furniture store. He had no experience in health care. One of the board members was his father-in-law, which explained how he got his job. He replaced Mr. Quinn Browning, who had retired that year.

Martin Gesso said to us, "The hospital administration has selected Dr. Brad Badger to be next year's chief of staff. We feel that Dr. Badger will faithfully protect the interests of the administration. The health care providers must accept that they will not be represented at the management level in the coming year. No questions will be permitted this evening."

Dr. Donald Strann, the current chief of staff, rose to ask a question anyway. "Mr. Gesso, are you aware of the fact that you are in violation of the hospital bylaws? The bylaws clearly state that the chief of staff is to be elected by a majority vote of the attending physicians currently having active privileges. Are you telling the medical staff that you intend to ignore the bylaws in the coming year?"

Gesso had no response to Strann's question. He had expected to ram his newly acquired authority down our throats without opposition. He did not know Donald Strann as well as I did.

Strann had delivered a big body blow. The board members glanced uncomfortably at each other with looks of disbelief. They squirmed in their seats and took sips of water.

"Mr. Gesso, we have patients to see," Strann said. "We can't sit here all night staring at each other. Please answer my question."

Gesso had no choice but to acknowledge that Strann was justified in citing the bylaws, and Gesso agreed to a paper ballot. Someone nominated Strann for reelection. When the votes were counted, Strann was reelected chief of staff by a margin of one vote. That evening the staff had bifurcated into two opposing camps, the sycophants and the rest of us. The latter group would henceforth be enemies of the state.

I, of course, had voted for Strann. He had done a good job as chief of staff, while Brad Badger had been divisive and abrasive. Badger was a general practitioner who hated and envied the specialists. He was delusional if he thought I would vote for him.

Gesso had sent a message that evening: he wanted the general staff to submit to his will. He did not want our input. We were to join lockstep with his agenda if we wished to survive at WGH. We had narrowly defeated him that evening, but it looked like we had a long year ahead of us.

I was not surprised when Brad Badger showed himself to be a sore loser. As each of the specialists exited the auditorium, he said to them, "You guys are going to live to regret this day."

October 16, 1997

Donald Strann, a respected medical oncologist, came to my office the morning after the staff meeting. I had the results of the previous day's computed tomography (CT) studies on his patients. Don had a busy schedule and I always conveyed information to him as concisely as possible. He virtually never engaged me in casual conversation, even though my wife, Joanie, worked for him as an oncology nurse. This morning, however, he took a seat in my office and accepted my offer of a cup of coffee.

"Tim, did you hear about the fistfight after the staff meeting?" he asked me.

"No, Don, I did not receive that particular information."

"Jim Rowley beat up Al Blank in Jim's office. Al ended up in the ER with broken ribs and facial contusions. As you probably know, those guys hate each other."

Jim Rowley was a private practice pediatrician who also served as the director of medical education (DME). Al Blank was a hospital-employed general practitioner who had already declared his loyalty to the new administration.

"Al followed Jim into his office and accused him of orchestrating the staff to reject Badger as chief of staff," Don explained. "Jim denied that he was involved, and they had an argument. Jim had an expensive ornamental porcelain rhinoceros on his desk. It was a present from the parents of a child Jim had cured of meningitis last year. I think the family was from Thailand, and it was a great honor for Jim to receive the gift. Anyway, the rhinoceros ended up in pieces on the floor as a result of Al knocking it off of Jim's desk, either deliberately or accidentally, depending on whom you believe. Jim lost his temper and beat the shit out of Al."

"My God," I replied. "By the way, congratulations about being reelected chief of staff last night. I was really concerned about Gesso and his little attempt at a coup. I'm really glad that you stood up to those assholes."

"Jim is on administrative leave pending further investigation," Don continued. "Al has been telling administration that this incident proves that some of the specialists are mentally unstable."

Naturally, within five minutes the radiologists converged on Gabe Watson's office. Gabe had been chairman of the department during the entire ten years I had been at WGH. After we rehashed the hideous details of Jim Rowley's pugilistic adventure, Gabe informed us of a problem in our own department. A particularly lazy technologist had boasted to Gabe that Martin Gesso had told him the techs should take every opportunity to file complaints about the radiologists. The tech had told Gabe that the rads would need to "watch ourselves." Gabe had not seen the humor in the tech's remark. He wanted to retaliate by cancelling the Christmas party we gave the techs every year to show our appreciation.

I agreed with Gabe and suggested that we make clear to the techs whom the offending individual was. The three other radiologists—Mike Morris, Phil Carlson, and Bob Percy—thought that it was unfair to punish all of the techs because of one person's stupidity. I could tell from Gabe's face that he was not to be deterred. He asserted his status as chairman and announced that the party would not happen this year.

I returned to my workstation in the CT department, where I was director. I enjoyed this responsibility, as the CT techs did high-quality work and were fun to be around. They got paid more than the general techs since they'd had additional training. As a result, the general techs hated the CT techs. They also hated and resented the radiologists because of our vastly greater income and status. They would hate us even more when they learned we'd cancelled their Christmas party.

Phil came into my office at the end of the afternoon. He had joined our group three years earlier, straight out of completing our residency program.

"The general techs have started acting like they own the department," he said. "They are complaining about everything I ask them to do. They are supposed to do what I tell them to do. It shouldn't be like this."

Our conversation was interrupted by the overhead intercom system.

"Code blue, administrative offices. Code blue, administrative offices. Code blue, administrative offices."

"I think I just want to be a radiologist for ten years." Phil went on. "When I have enough money, I want to quit medicine and run a fishing boat operation in Key West."

"Phil, a code blue has been called in the administrative offices," I said. That meant someone's heart had stopped beating. After a few minutes, one of the CT techs informed me that we had received an order for an emergency head CT on the stricken individual. She said we would be ready to receive the patient in five minutes.

Neurosurgeon Dr. Vincent Gustavo appeared in my office. Vince told me that the person whose heart had stopped beating was Dr. John Dodson, a WGH obstetrician.

"Tim, John was just starting a deposition in a malpractice case when he collapsed," Vince said. "His blood pressure was sky high. He had no heart activity and no respirations. The code team intubated him and got his heart started. I did a quick neurological exam on him. I am certain he had a massive intracranial bleed. I need a head CT to confirm my diagnosis."

"Vince, that is so sad. Look, I need to go help the techs get John in the scanner."

We gently placed John in the CT gantry and carefully positioned his head in the aperture of the scanner. After ninety seconds of scanning and thirty seconds of data processing, we began to receive images of his brain. The elapsed time from starting the scan to confirming Vince's clinical diagnosis was three minutes. John would be taken to the ICU and given medicine to control his blood pressure and reduce brain swelling.

Vince followed me into my office. "Tim, several years ago John performed a delivery that didn't turn out well. As you know, all of us who practice medicine long enough will eventually have something bad happen. The plaintiff's attorney was just peppering John with hostile questions. John is a sensitive person and I think it was too much for him. His wife is on her way to the ICU."

I finally finished my work and went home. I felt very stressed out by the events of the week, though I thought my stress level was probably miniscule compared to doctors like Vince and John. It had always been easy for me to understand why physicians were so vulnerable to developing substance abuse problems. It almost came with the job description.

Joanie would be home any minute. I was looking forward to simply having dinner and watching TV.

Joanie and I had been introduced to each other by a mutual friend at a hospital social event. Even though Joanie had worked at Strann's office for many years, our paths had never crossed previously, since Strann's office was an outpatient clinic. Joanie only rarely had a need to visit the hospital. After we were introduced, the rest, as they say, was history. We had been married for three years.

"I'm home," Joanie called from the hallway.

I turned the television off and greeted Joanie in the kitchen. I put our dinner in the microwave. We would be having leftover lasagna.

"Did you just get home?" Joanie asked.

"About twenty minutes ago."

I told her about John Dodson's collapse. Many of our graphic evening discussions would not have appealed to most people, but they were completely natural for us.

"How was work?" I asked.

"It was busy, as usual. Patient-wise, everything was fine. We had our pipeline meeting to discuss next week's treatment plans. After pipeline, Strann and Furst had an argument about the plans for our new office building."

She changed the subject. "I want to shave the cats tonight, give them a lion's cut. They have been licking themselves all the time. Jasper has been vomiting fur balls every night. Will you hold them down while I shave them?"

"Sure, no problem. Let's eat dinner, shave the cats, and then watch some TV. I think *The X-Files* is on tonight."

# Chapter 3

Joanie was thirty-eight years old in 1997, very attractive, with short blond hair and blue eyes. When we first met, I was immediately attracted to her voice. She has a lovely voice and is a talented singer. She performs with a band at local weddings.

I was forty-six years old then, with brown eyes and brown hair. I have an average height and build. I like to read and exercise. I especially like to run, swim, and ride my road bike. I have participated in a few short-course triathlons, though with only modest results. My reading tastes are protean. I will read almost any genre except for romance novels and science fiction. I also enjoy listening to classical music.

I try very hard to live a normal life. It is possible, although not easy, to be a balanced and mentally healthy person while being a physician. Many of us could be accurately described as borderline, or actual, sociopaths. As a group we tend to be moody, obsessive compulsive, chronically depressed, and egotistical. I occasionally had these tendencies. I never delved into the details of what I did at the hospital with other people. Much of what I saw and did would have been disturbing to most people. This made me feel isolated from other people. I think most physicians feel isolated.

I was lucky to have Joanie to talk to. Not every woman would have placed the above qualities in the plus column of their score sheets when seeking a mate. However, Joanie had been a nurse for twelve years. She knew that most physicians were not exactly poster children when it came to mental health. She would jokingly tell me that physicians suffered from a combination of Asperger's and Tourette's syndromes.

I should speak briefly of my background. I became attracted to the field of medicine early in my undergraduate studies. Like all undergraduates, I needed to figure out if there was anything I was particularly good at. My only real strength was science. Like most pre-med students, I didn't know much about the practical realities of the medical profession. I just thought I wanted to be a physician. Besides, I couldn't think of anything else to do with my life.

I might have tried to become a philosophy professor if the job prospects had been better. I was fascinated by philosophy, even though I was not a particularly brilliant student of the subject. Nevertheless, I wanted to learn as much as I could about the "great thinkers," both ancient and modern. I ended up graduating with a double major in pre-medical studies and philosophy. After graduation, I attended medical school. More about my background later.

$Chapter$ **4**

---

October 18, 1997

The rads were holding a meeting in Gabe's office. John Dodson's condition had deteriorated and the life support systems had been withdrawn. He never regained consciousness. His funeral was to be held on October 22. This morning the malpractice attorney had called the hospital to find out when John could continue his deposition.

"These people come from another planet," I said to the group. "Here we have this poor man dying in the ICU and all the attorney cares about is when he can resume his hourly billing."

Gabe informed us that Jim Rowley was forced to resign as director of medical education (DME) as a result of having beat up Al
Blank. A replacement DME had not yet been found. Gabe also
warned us that the news of the cancellation of the techs' Christmas
party had spread through the department. The techs would be
looking for reasons to complain about us to administration. We
needed to be careful in our dealings with the techs.

John Dodson's funeral was held at Christ Catholic Church, several blocks from the hospital. I went to the funeral to represent
the radiology department. We had sent a wreath and contributed
money to the John Dodson Memorial Fund. The church was filled
to capacity.

I had known John fairly well and liked him immensely. He was
always kind to everyone. He had often told me that what my office
needed was a window. I appreciated that he related to me on a
personal level instead of just being concerned about test results.

A close church friend of John's delivered the eulogy. I will
always remember the following part. John's friend said, "You learn
a lot about a man by being out with him on his boat. John loved his
sailboat. One day we were out sailing, and John told me what was
important to him in life. The important things to John were his
family and his belief in God. The community will deeply mourn
the passing of this fine and decent man."

Although the medical staff were deeply affected by John's
death, the contrast between the church and medical communities
was obvious to me. Doctors get back to business very quickly. They
do not dwell for very long on the passing or retirement of a colleague. The reality is that we really did not know very much about
each other.

However, a colleague of John's in the obstetrics department,
Dr. Leo Sandusky, was present at the funeral. He had been asked
to speak to the congregation.

"John Dodson was a fine obstetrician and a compassionate
man," he said. "He was always calm and reassuring, even in the
most stressful situations. He remembered the names of all of his
patients and their families, and not only his current patients. John
passed away far too early in his life, but he achieved a standard of

living and practicing medicine that all physicians should aspire to. I am proud to have been associated with John."

After the eulogies, we formed a line to offer words of consolation to John's widow, Lily. I had never met Lily before. I mentioned to her that I had played a small part in caring for John.

"Mrs. Dodson, I know that John did not suffer," I said. "All of us loved and respected him. He was one of the finest men I have ever known."

"Dr. Duncan, did you say you were at the hospital when John died?"

"Yes, Mrs. Dodson, I was in the radiology department when John was starting to give his deposition."

"Dr. Duncan, the malpractice lawyer called John's lawyer and told him they are not going to drop the suit against John. He wants to go after John's estate. I haven't slept since John collapsed."

"Lily, I doubt that they can continue the suit. John never completed his deposition. Besides, there is always John's malpractice insurance."

"But the malpractice lawyer said they would go after both the insurance company and the estate."

"Lily, please listen carefully. These people come from another planet. They have no scruples. Even as you grieve, they are trying to scare you into pressuring the insurance company to throw money at them in order to protect John's estate. Whatever you do, don't panic. They are simply trying to frighten you. The things that some lawyers do sicken me. Listen to your lawyer. He will protect John's estate."

_Chapter_ **5**

A radiologist would not need to conduct a national survey or consult a think tank to understand the tremendous influence the threat of lawsuits has on the way physicians practice medicine. Almost all physicians practice defensive medicine. I saw it every day at WGH. Doctors order expensive diagnostic tests and procedures that have little potential benefit to the patient in order to protect themselves from litigation. I would never criticize them for ordering these unnecessary tests. They are not being paranoid. Physicians are never sued for ordering too many tests. The basis for many lawsuits is that a physician withheld a test, even when he or she had good reasons for doing so.

Doctors are sometimes accused of overusing these tests and procedures in order to become wealthy. This allegation may have validity when the physician has a financial interest in the equipment used to perform the test. In my case, however, the hospital owned all of the imaging equipment. I got paid by the insurance companies. Our referring doctors had no financial incentive to overprescribe my services. In fact, many of them were somewhat resentful of the financial rewards radiologists received from scanning large numbers of patients. Physicians were not ordering excessive radiology services so that radiologists could drive expensive cars. They were ordering these services to protect themselves from frivolous lawsuits.

What is the correct or ideal number of CT scans that should be ordered per thousand patient visits to the ER? No one knows the answer to that question. What is known is that there is a wide variation among individual ER physicians. It is generally accepted that there is an eightfold variation in the number of CT scans ordered between the highest and lowest utilizers. The only way to roughly assess an individual ER physician's rate of ordering CT scans is to compare him to his peers. Some hospital organizations have begun to collect utilization data and to inform physicians how they compare to their peers. This data is not intended as a criticism, since there are no reliable data to determine if patients suffer when fewer scans are ordered, or if they significantly benefit from a higher rate of utilization.

It seems logical that physicians might benefit in some way from knowing how they compare with their peers. But what happens when the entire composite group of ER physicians feels the need to practice defensive medicine to a greater or lesser degree? Determining the ideal absolute number of medically indicated studies becomes even harder to determine, since everyone is overusing these studies, to some extent, because of the fear of lawsuits. I realize that no one claims that comparison studies can determine the ideal rate of CT utilization if only medically indicated studies were ordered. However, I cannot help but speculate what would happen if, instead of comparing one fearful physician with another, someone did a study of utilization rates in an environment where nobody was afraid of being sued.

Studies that compare the utilization rates of other countries with the United States probably come closest to falling in this category. It is true that many more high-tech diagnostic studies are performed per capita in the United States than in any other country, and that these tests are an important reason why health care costs are so significant. But it is equally true that no other country in the world tolerates the number of frivolous lawsuits that are everyday occurrences in the United States—and not just of the medical malpractice variety. Spilling hot coffee on your lap will not make you and your lawyer multimillionaires anywhere except in the United States. The reason this can happen in the United States is political. The politicians in Washington receive enormous amounts of money from trial lawyers. And unless I have been misled by all of my reading on the subject, most of this money goes to Democrats.

Regardless of whether or not you believe that limits should be placed on the legal profession, it always annoys me when the issue of tort reform is ignored in discussions about the rising costs of health care (and it always is). It is obvious that the threat of medical malpractice lawsuits is a significant factor in driving up health care costs. The federal government has the power and the responsibility to pass legislation so that a patient who has been harmed by a medical mistake is fairly compensated, while at the same time placing restrictions on exorbitant awards that are not justified. And yet our elected leaders will continue to remain silent about tort reform.

*Chapter* **6**

The relationship between administration and the radiology department at WGH was a nurturing one during the first ten years of my tenure. The CEO of the hospital during that time, Mr. Quinn Browning, had great respect for physicians. His background was in education, but he always listened carefully to a doctor's opinion. He always collaborated with us. He never issued an ultimatum.

To give an example, one time the radiology department wanted a new ultrasound machine, and I was given the job of presenting our case. I met with Mr. Browning in his office and requested that the hospital allocate $300,000 to purchase a new machine. I explained that with an updated array of ultrasound transducers, we would dramatically improve our image quality. Further, we would insure that physicians continued to refer patients to us. Medical imaging is an intensely competitive business and imaging centers abounded in the city, all of us competing for a finite number of patients. By obtaining state-of-the-art equipment, we would improve patient care and at the same time increase our number of referrals in order to pay off the capital expenditure.

I was about to expound further to Mr. Browning when he interrupted me. "Dr. Duncan, you don't have to say another word. You have made your case. I will approve the purchase. The radiology department has never given me bad advice."

I thanked Mr. Browning for supporting my department. Our discussion had taken less than thirty minutes. The whole process had been as painless as an ultrasound examination is for our patients.

I became apprehensive when Mr. Browning retired on September 15, 1997. My department frequently needed new equipment. There would be a new CEO and a new administration. Would these new guys be responsive to our needs?

*Chapter* 7

October 29, 1997

We in the radiology department decided we might as well find out sooner rather than later how responsive the new administration was. We needed a nuclear medicine single-photon emission computed tomography (SPECT) camera. This technology is essential for a noninvasive evaluation of cardiac blood flow. The cardiologists considered the test to be a vital component in their evaluation of patients with chest pain.

Once again I was assigned the job of getting approval for the purchase. I found myself sitting in a walnut-tabled conference room with four executive vice presidents whom I had never met. I began my presentation. "Gentlemen, thank you for meeting with me. My name is Dr. Duncan and I represent the radiology department. I have come to you to request that the hospital allocate $200,000 for the purchase of a SPECT camera for our nuclear medicine department. The camera is essential for cardiac imaging. Every day, the cardiologists are currently sending out four patients with chest pain to other hospitals because we lack a SPECT camera. If we retain those four patients a day, we should be able to pay off the camera in eighteen months."

George Gravy, executive vice president of financial affairs, asked, "Doctor, are you aware that health care is a business?"

"Mr. Gravy, I recognize that, in certain respects, health care is a business. I am glad you brought this subject up. My department makes about $9 million a year for the hospital. We generate more revenue by far than any other department. So we feel that, from a business perspective, it makes sense to invest in the radiology department. By the way, most people call me Dr. Duncan. I do have a name."

"Doctor, you are telling us this camera costs $200,000?"

"Our preliminary investigation with equipment manufacturers indicates a price in that range."

"So you have already spoken to these companies without first consulting with administration?"

"Of course we have. We know the prices of all the equipment we may need in the future."

"Doctor, don't you already have enough toys? Your request is not consistent with cost containment. Or didn't they teach you about cost containment in medical school?" The executive vice presidents enjoyed a good chuckle among themselves.

"The cardiologists don't consider the camera to be a toy," I said. "They consider it to be a way they can tell if a patient is having a heart attack. Here, let me give you copies of a letter they wrote in support of this purchase."

The vice presidents barely glanced at the letter. Then Mr. Gravy stood and indicated the meeting was over. "Doctor, we will consider your request," he said. "But if I were you, I would not hold my breath."

I immediately called a meeting of the radiologists and told them about Gravy's remarks. "I felt like I was point man in a parallel universe. They just eviscerated me. These new guys don't know the first thing about medicine and they don't want to learn. Thank goodness we got most of our equipment updated before Browning left. These guys aren't going to give us the time of day."

"Tim, you did the best you could," said my colleague Phil. "Maybe the cardiologists can put pressure on these guys. Maybe Peter Murphy can convince them to buy the camera."

"Yeah," I said. "And maybe I will play for the Red Wings next year."

Chapter 8

The practice of medicine, like much of life, can be dull and mundane. One way we tried to alleviate the boredom was our weekly "interesting case conference," when we educated our two residents as we discussed particularly interesting or educational cases. One week I grilled Casey Price, who was in his second year of our four-year program.

"Dr. Price," I began, in the decades-long tradition of medical education, "you are presented with an X-ray of the left ankle in a nineteen-year-old patient. Please describe the findings."

"We have a standard three-view study of the left ankle," he answered. "There appears to be a fracture—"

"No, Casey," I interrupted. "You always want to sound decisive in everything you say. I want you to remove the word 'appears' from your vocabulary from now on. Tell me that there is a fracture."

My teaching style resembled *The Gong Show*—I'd let a resident keep talking until he made a mistake. Then the hook came out and he was "gonged." Casey started over.

"There is an oblique fracture through the distal fibula which is mildly displaced and angulated."

This was good stuff, so I encouraged Casey by asking him questions. "Is the fracture through normal bone?"

"No, the underlying bone is not normal. There is an abnormal lucency in the bone."

"Wonderful. Casey, now tell me more about the lucency. Is it central or eccentric? Does it expand the bone? Does it have a matrix—meaning, is there any density within the center of the lucency?"

"It is expansile, eccentric, and has a swirly central matrix."

"Excellent. Do you have a diagnosis?"

"Yes, I have a diagnosis. This is a pathologic fracture through a non-ossifying fibroma, which is a benign tumor of bone."

"Very good, Casey. Do you see how easy it is to make a correct diagnosis when you describe the findings correctly?"

Of course, it was not always this easy. This was a fairly obvious case. But I always tried to build up our residents' confidence. I will always remember when one of my colleagues described the radiology reports as "often wrong but never in doubt." It was a funny line, but not entirely accurate, as I'm sure he knew. We did in fact have doubts about some cases. But while it was true that we were wrong sometimes, with the correct approach we were rarely grossly incorrect, although I suppose that happened to all radiologists once in a while. It takes a lot of confidence to deal with ambiguity, and we all make an occasional mistake. Radiologists, like all physicians, must learn to not let their mistakes bother them too much. Mistakes must be seen as learning experiences. In medical school they taught us to "forgive yourself, but remember."

I further explained to Casey, "The analytic process usually occurs only in the mind of an experienced radiologist. Our referring doctors care more about the final diagnosis, which is found at the conclusion of the report. At these weekly confer- ences, however, we need to talk about the analytic process so that you learn the correct concepts."

I always enjoyed having residents in the department. I liked to teach. It made me feel good to contribute to their education. They provided good company, and we usually ended up being good friends. They provided relief from most of the "scut work."

However, there was a considerable danger in training residents. We were producing a young talent pool which lacked "street smarts" and economic leverage. When they finished their training, a hospital could try to hire the young guns, pay them well below their worth, and replace the existing radiologists. We were potentially train- ing our own competition. Most of our residents would never have betrayed us this way, but you never knew about everyone.

One of our defenses against this would have been to hire our residents as soon as they finished their training and to exploit them ourselves. Another common strategy was to abuse them so badly during their residency that they wanted to get as far away from us as possible when they graduated. This was a good way to create a radiologic diaspora. Personally, I did not advocate these approaches. My ethical imperative, as much as I might have been in the minority, was to treat residents and small animals humanely.

The so-called RAPE specialists (radiologists, anesthesiologists, pathologists, and emergency room) were particularly vulnerable to being thrown out and replaced by our graduating residents. The reason for this was to be found in the much-loved and much- hated "exclusive contract" the RAPE specialists usually had to sign with the hospital. The much-loved "exclusive" part meant that only the radiologists of that particular group could bill insurance companies for studies performed using the hospital's equipment. We were less thrilled with the "contract" part, which provided that a hostile administration could threaten to not renew our contract at the end of three years should we not comply with their hideous intentions.

The common denominator among RAPE specialists was that we occupied the physical space of the hospital. In addition, our equipment was expensive. Since most of us were not multimillionaires, the hospital owned the equipment we need to perform our jobs. The radiologists at WGH were currently working under the "fee for service" arrangement. The insurance companies paid us a set fee for each study we interpreted, and paid the hospital a "technical" fee to offset the costs of the equipment and to pay for their walnut-tabled conference rooms. There was a rough inverse correlation between the quality of the carpet in the administrative offices and the degree of dilapidation in our scanning equipment. In a typical fee-for-service arrangement, the hospital technical fee was about twice as large as the radiologists' interpretation fee. We always told our colleagues that when the radiologists did well, the hospital did twice as well. In other words, the administration had no legitimate reason to bitch about the current arrangement.

Since we were the first letter in the RAPE acronym, we were always worried that the new administration would try to kill the golden-egg-laying goose. They could demand that we become hospital employees at our next contract renewal. The hospital would collect both of the fees from the insurance companies, while throwing us a tiny bone in the form of a miniscule monthly paycheck. This abomination had already come to fruition in the pathology department. We rads had spread the word that any attempt by admin to impose this arrangement with us would result in a scorched-earth response in which we would all resign. We knew we could live for about a year on the income from services already rendered. The immediate revenues of the hospital would not increase one dime if we all resigned. They would have a hard time recruiting quality radiologists on salary. If they expected a high-quality radiologist to come to the hospital, they would probably have to agree to a fee-for-service contract. So they would end up in the same place as we were currently, provided the hospital did not go bankrupt while they were trying to recruit our replacements. The situation reminded me of the post–World War II strategy of "mutual assured destruction" (MAD). Of course, the inherent danger of MAD was that some deranged madman could decide to push the red button. There was no shortage of such people in the new administration.

$Chapter$ **9**

## November 20, 1997

I left work at noon. Each rad was given a half-day off each week, and today was mine. I filled my car with gas, purchased some groceries, and jogged my three-mile course at a local park. Then I went home to shower. There was a visualization I always used in the shower. I imagined my body to have been sprayed with a continuous stream of granular, toxic waste material at work all week. There was a chance I could survive another week at WGH if I could wash away this toxic material at a rate greater than its accretion. Seth Davis, anesthesiologist, had explained this process to me as a dynamic equilibrium. According to his theory, the shit flowed in and the shit flowed out. If the rates of shit inflow and outflow were equal, we would not drown in the shit. Our primary goal must always be to keep our heads above the shit level.

Seth knew what he was talking about. As an anesthesiologist, the specialty I considered to be the most important, he was frequently subjected to abuse. Surgeons taking a breather from removing a hydroptic gall bladder seemed to find that it relieved stress to verbally abuse the anesthesiologist. The surgeons at WGH considered other physicians to be subordinate planets revolving around the scalpel-wielding sun. We were unworthy to receive the surgeon's life-giving illumination. Seth was frequently exposed to a solar flare.

This particular day I had dinner to prepare, so I knew I needed to stop this internal conversation. I dried myself off and put on my sweat clothes. I went into the kitchen to start dinner. Our cats, Jasper and Cala, were sunning themselves on the kitchen counter. I would gladly have traded job descriptions with either of them.

Joanie came home an hour later and we sat down to eat.

"Are you going to use your telescope tonight?" she asked.

I shook my head. "It will be too cloudy. I'll look at Jupiter tomorrow night if it clears up. I need to build a plywood platform with wheels on the bottom so I can roll the damn thing out onto the back patio instead of herniating myself carrying it out there."

Phil Carson and I had recently decided we would each buy an eight-inch reflecting telescope and become amateur astronomers. We would compare our nightly observations over breakfast in the doctors' dining room. I had subscribed to *Astronomy Today* magazine.

This seemed to me to be an excellent hobby. So far I had enjoyed using my telescope, except for the evening I was out on the driveway in front of our house and a police car drove up because a neighbor said I was trying to observe her naked body through her bathroom window as she was preparing to take a shower. After I showed the policeman the nebula in Orion's belt, he drove off without arresting me.

# Chapter 10

November 22, 1997

Casey Price and I were working out of my office. Casey was amusing me with stories about the citywide residents' conference he had attended over the weekend. I sipped coffee from a mug that said "Radiologists do it in the dark." I couldn't remember how I obtained the mug, but I was going to get rid of it. Someone might charge me with sexual harassment if they saw it.

One of our nuclear medicine techs, Allison West, came into my office. "Dr. Duncan, we have a problem. An older gentleman who claims he is a hospital VIP is in the department and is freaking out. He says his wife is having chest pain and the cardiologist is telling him we can't take care of her at Wilno General, that she needs to be transferred across town."

"Allison, I will come right over, but first do me a favor and find out this gentleman's name." I turned to Casey. "I think we have a developing situation on our hands."

Allison soon returned to inform us that the gentleman's name was Mr. Gravy.

"My God," I said. The three of us trooped across the hall to find that George Gravy, executive vice president of financial affairs, was indeed in the department and that he was highly agitated.

"What is the meaning of this?" Gravy ranted. "Who is in charge here? I am a hospital VIP and my wife is having chest pain. She may be having a heart attack, for God's sake!"

I spoke patiently, savoring every word. "Who is in charge here would be me. My name is Dr. Duncan, in case you forgot. The reason we cannot care for your wife at Wilno General is because we do not have a SPECT camera. If I recall correctly, I had a meeting with you last month and requested that the hospital purchase a SPECT camera. At the end of the meeting, you told me not to hold my breath. Mr. Gravy, I have not been holding my breath. I trust that your wife will receive excellent care at another hospital. And by the way, *this* is the kind of thing they teach us at medical school."

This was not Mr. Gravy's finest hour. He had just been dressed down by a physician. His face assumed a peculiar cyanotic hue. I did not rule out the possibility of a husband-wife combo cardiac event. After we took his blood pressure, I concluded he was having a harmless vasovagal reaction. His life was not in danger, but I had the tech take him to the ER as a precaution.

Six weeks later we installed our SPECT camera.

$$Chapter\ 11$$

Christmas Eve, 1997

The Christmas dinner for the radiologists and residents, together with our wives or significant others, was held at the downtown Wilno Four Seasons hotel. I was on call that evening, so I would not be drinking any alcohol. Sparkling water would have to suffice. I don't really drink a lot of alcohol anyway. We were all seated in a private dining room. Gabe Watson enjoyed fine food and cognac, and when we had a party during his tenure as chairman, he spared no expense. Tonight we were celebrating the passing of another year in which none of us had grossly embarrassed the department with scandal, sexual impropriety, illicit drug abuse, or general mayhem.

Gabe stood to address the group. "Tonight we celebrate the achievements of the year. We appreciate the hard work of our residents. All things considered, it was a good year. Our numbers improved over last year's. I know that all of us are under a lot of pressure. All of you guys did an outstanding job. I want to toast to our having many more successful years."

We all raised our glasses in acknowledgement of Gabe's leadership. As we sat down to order our dinners, I checked my beeper to make sure the batteries were fully charged. I did this every hour that my beeper remained silent. Joanie and I were seated between Gabe and his wife, Diane, on our left, and Casey and his girlfriend, Stephanie, on our right. Casey and I were doing impersonations of our least favorite referring doctors. Halfway through our salads, Gabe turned to me and dropped his bombshell.

"Tim, I am considering stepping down as chairman. The group needs new blood, maybe someone who can work better with the new administration. They are already pissed off at me."

I didn't want Gabe to step down and I told him so. "Gabe, I'm not sure I want someone who can work better with administration, considering their agenda. They are going to be pissed off at anyone who won't kiss their asses. You've been chairman for ten years and you have done a great job. You have connections and histories with guys in all kinds of departments that none of us have. There could be unintended consequences if you step down. Besides, as far as I know, none of us really wants to be chairman."

At that time we bestowed the chairman with a stipend of $10,000 a year as compensation for the worthless meetings he had to attend while the rest of us played racquetball at the Michigan Athletic Club, or slept. We could have raised the stipend, but I knew money was not the issue for Gabe. Maybe he was just tired of being chairman. I needed to change the subject.

"Gabe, how is the karate coming along? I notice you have facial contusions." This injury was small potatoes compared to the metacarpal fractures, cervical hematomas, and auricular lacerations Gabe had suffered in the past. Dr. Mark Casper, WGH neurologist and Gabe's regular sparring partner, had once explained the intense pleasure he derived from planting his fully extended heel onto Gabe's hard palate, even as Gabe broke Mark's nose.

"I took second place at our regional competition," Gabe said. "Mark only took fifth."

Joanie and I finished our dinners well ahead of the others. Since I was on call, I needed to get home in order to be close to the hospital when the DUI car crashes started. Besides, the weather was deteriorating. We collected our car from valet parking and headed home.

# Chapter 12

## January 10, 1998

We were required to accumulate one hundred and fifty hours of continuing medical education (CME) every three years in order to maintain our state medical licenses. I carefully documented the lectures I attended or gave, journal articles I read, and the medical audiotapes I listened to on the way to work and coming home. Fifty of the hours had to be "category one," which were obtained by attending a conference accredited by the American College of Radiology. Our corporation provided each of us with a yearly stipend of five thousand dollars to attend conferences. This amount of money easily covered one conference a year. I was able to stretch my money to cover two conferences a year by being frugal in my choice of hotel accommodations. I attended an extra conference a year because, in addition to staying current in my specialty areas, I was learning a new modality: magnetic resonance imaging (MRI).

I always attended the winter conference presented by Stanford University in Snowmass, Colorado. At the 1998 conference the morning session of lectures ran from seven to eleven. We got a few hours off to ski, and then we returned for the afternoon sessions, which ran from four to seven. I would obtain twenty-five hours of credit for the week.

The radiology conference coincided with the Harvard University Pathology Conference, also in Snowmass. A colleague of mine at WGH, pathologist Fred Quimby, always attended this conference with his wife, Karen. The three of us would ski together most days. Fred wore his long gray hair in a ponytail. Fred and Karen were better skiers than I, but they would patiently wait for me to catch up with them because we were good friends.

Thursday night we were eating dinner at a German restaurant in downtown Snowmass, a short shuttle ride from our hotels. At the end of the meal, I was enjoying a piece of German chocolate cake, my favorite dessert. Fred and Karen each had an apple strudel in front of them. I said to Fred, "I have two questions for you. First, what do you think of our new administration, and second, what did you learn at your conference?"

"To answer your first question," Fred began, "Gesso is going to run the hospital like a dictatorship. He has already told me to cut my hair. I felt like we were back in high school. He can go fuck himself. I am not going to cut my hair. That reminds me—somebody, probably Brad Badger, told him I used the F-word in the doctors' dining room. Gesso told me to clean up my language. Tim, Gesso will want to force you guys to become hospital employees. Take it from me, you don't want to let that happen. The pathologists agreed to become employees a few years ago, and it was the stupidest thing we have ever done. Quinn Browning treated us fairly well, but these new guys are a different story. We will never get a raise. They are going to tell us how much vacation time we can take. I wish I had enough money to retire, but I don't.

"To answer your second question, there was a lecture about the human papilloma virus, HPV, and how it may be related to the development of cervical cancer. The rest of the lectures were pretty unremarkable. How about your conference?"

I told Fred about a noteworthy lecture concerning a new, safer intravenous contrast agent that had been developed for radiologic studies. It was widely known that the agent we were using was generally safe, but one in forty thousand contrast injections resulted in a fatal allergic reaction. The newer agent was about twice as safe, but it cost five times as much as the older agent. This created a significant dilemma. We could restrict the use of the new agent to patients who had risk factors for a reaction, such as asthma, seafood allergies, and renal problems. However, fatal reactions could also occur in patients who had no risk factors. The other way to go was to use the new agent in all of our patients. This would raise the cost of the contrast agent for the hospital, and not all insurance companies were willing to reimburse the extra cost. I had started to get a headache by the end of this lecture. I could only imagine how this dilemma was going to play out at WGH. A lot of radiologists would have pretended that they had skipped this lecture, but that was not my way of doing things. Problems need to be confronted, not ignored.

The lecturer had reached the conclusion that we should all convert to the exclusive use of the new agent, in the interest of patient safety. He said that even though most of us had probably never had a patient death with the old agent, this would not justify our continuing to use it in the future. He used a joke to illustrate his point.

"A twelve-year-old girl tells her mother that she wants to marry her seventh grade sweetheart, Billy, and start a family. The mother explains to her daughter that babies cost a lot of money, and that it is important for girls to protect themselves from becoming pregnant before they are married. The girl tells her mother, 'Yes, Billy and I will not have a baby before we are married. But we figure so far, so good.'"

It occurred to me that this was the same punch line as the reply given by the man who, having jumped off the roof of a twenty-story building, was asked how he was doing as he passed the eighteenth floor.

A radiologist in the audience had asked the lecturer how he could convince his hospital administration to pay the extra cost, when he was having trouble even getting them to replace the light bulbs in his view box. The lecturer had said that the only way to do this was to send a certified letter to administration to inform them that a safer agent was available. This would create "shared responsibility." In the lexicon of people everywhere, this meant CYA—cover your ass.

$$\mathscr{C}hapter\ \mathbf{13}$$

Upon my return to WGH from the winter conference, I told the other rads about the new contrast agent. I wanted to send a certified letter to our administration. I offered to write and send it, but I stipulated that I wanted all of us to sign it. All of the rads refused. I sent the letter anyway, affixed with my solitary signature. I had no qualms about it. I took patient safety very seriously. It simply made no sense to pretend there was no problem. We would have to switch to the new agent eventually, so why wait until there was a patient death, when it would be too late?

Administration's reaction to my letter, of which I of course had kept a copy, was thermonuclear. Gesso called Gabe and told him

I was a "loose cannon." How could I put such a recommendation in writing? I had created a "paper trail," for God's sake.

Of course, that had been the whole point of the letter. Absent that letter, I knew exactly how the administration would handle the situation if we had a patient death. We would be sued for tens of millions of dollars. The hospital representative would testify in his deposition, "We were never told by the radiologists that there was a safer agent. Frankly, I am surprised they were taking such chances with patient safety, apparently just to save money. We would have gladly paid the extra cost for the new agent if we had been told it was available. We are going to cancel their contract. It is inexcusable for them to keep using the old agent without consulting us."

There was no way I was going to let that happen, even though I knew the other rads did not support me. One of the great philosophers said that the most dangerous thing a person could be was "ahead of his time." While the other rads were probably not going to burn me at the stake, I was starting to feel like a wounded calf in *Wild Kingdom*, watching the herd abandon me to my fate at the hand, or paw, of the stalking lion.

At the next rad meeting, Gabe said to me, "Tim, the administration is very upset about the letter you sent them."

"Oh, really?" I said. "Excuse me for not being surprised. When have they ever provided a helpful response to a legitimate problem? It is not my fault that there is a safer contrast agent, and that using it is the new standard of care. I'm just the messenger. You guys might not care about patient safety, but I do. Mike, if your wife or kids needed a contrast injection, would you use the safest agent?"

"Of course I would."

"But you would use the old agent if the patient was a stranger?"

"Yes."

"Isn't that hypocritical?"

"No."

"Isn't that being hypocritical about being hypocritical? Isn't that hypocrisy squared?"

"No."

"This discussion could lead to an infinite regress of being hypocritical."

"Tim, you have to look at the whole picture. You need to consider administration's point of view."

"Gabe, they don't have a point of view for me to consider. Attacking me does not represent a point of view about the contrast issue. Look, we are getting nowhere here. I wrote the letter, which buys all of us some protection. By the way, you guys could have just said the issue needs further evaluation."

"The issue does need further evaluation."

"Thank you."

As it turned out, we did not need to evaluate the issue much further. The day after our meeting, a twenty-year-old man had a severe contrast reaction that was nearly fatal. All of the contrast media were removed from the department, to be replaced by the new agent. No one said a word to me about the sudden change in policy.

*Chapter* **14**

October is Breast Cancer Awareness Month. But for some reason, a local television station wanted to run a segment about breast cancer in April of 1998. They wanted to film an interview with one of us about screening mammograms. Although none of us in the department were grossly disfigured, we all had some disqualifying characteristic—I had a tendency to mumble sometimes, for example. All of us, that is, except for Mike Morris, who had a good understanding of breast cancer issues and was quite articulate. We decided he should give the interview. I watched the taped segment at home.

Mike was asked to explain why it was important for women to receive yearly screening mammograms, beginning at the age of forty.

Mike explained, "It is important because the rate of cure of breast cancer is directly related to the size of the cancer at the time of diagnosis and treatment. The cure rate when the cancer is the size of a raisin or smaller approaches 90 percent. When the cancer is the size of a walnut, the cure rate is reduced to about 50 percent. Most small cancers cannot be detected by physical examination, although monthly self-examinations are still an important part of detection. Mammograms are safe and affordable. The discomfort from compression of the breasts is acceptable to almost all of our patients."

Discomfort is a relative term, of course. Most of us radiologists referred to the test as a "slammogram," on occasion, but we are only joking. The techs were trained to keep patient discomfort to a minimum.

The interviewer asked Steve to comment on the criticism that benign masses were sometimes biopsied, and that some cancers were not detected by mammography.

"Those concerns are valid," Mike acknowledged. "Sometimes we cannot be certain that a solid mass is benign unless we obtain a small tissue sample using a very fine needle. Such biopsies are virtually painless and never cause any disfigurement of the breast.

"It is also true that about 10 percent of cancers are invisible on mammograms, because they are obscured or hiding in normal but dense glandular tissue. This means that we can never prove unequivocally that a woman does not have cancer. The value of the test is that it does detect 90 percent of cancers."

Mike had done a good job. Those of us involved in the diagnosis and treatment of breast cancer wanted women to be fully educated about this deadly disease. Even now, a lot of what is reported by the media is false and misleading. The truth is that mammograms save lives.

I cornered Mike in his office the following day.

"Hey, Mikey, you looked great on television last night. It is amazing what they can do with makeup these days."

Mike replied affably, "Hey, Tim, bite me."

*Chapter* **15**

Gabe decided to resign from the chairmanship in April of 1998.

Gabe and I had been at WGH for ten years. Before WGH, I worked at a small community hospital in eastern Pennsylvania. I had completed my fellowship training in CT scanning and interventional radiology (IR) and had passed my board examinations. I should have been happy, but there was a problem: I hated my job. The chairman of the department was a real jerk. He verbally abused everyone in the department. He was always playing golf while the rest of us slaved away at the hospital, and then he would complain about how lazy we all were. I didn't want to waste any more time at that job. I was looking for an opportunity to leave.

I was sitting at my work station on January 10, 1987, when I received the phone call that would provide me the chance to escape.

"This is Dr. Gabe Watson, calling from Wilno, Michigan. Is this Dr. Duncan?"

"Yes, you are speaking to Dr. Duncan. How are you, Dr. Watson? What can I do for you?"

"I am the chairman of the radiology department at Wilno General Hospital. I am going to form a new radiology department here. The old group was asked to leave. No one here knows how to read a CT scan. I am fellowship-trained in angiography. I got your name from Gene Seaver, who said he knows you from your residency program. I wanted to recruit Gene, but he is from Texas, and he doesn't want to freeze his ass off up here during the winter. I need an expert in CT scanning. Some interventional experience would be good but isn't necessary."

I had to be careful not to spill my coffee all over the $50,000 work station. I told Gabe I would be there the next week for an interview.

I took two days of vacation time and flew to Michigan. Gabe picked me up at the airport and brought me to his impressive house. We talked about our training and backgrounds. He took me to dinner that evening and told me some specifics. I would be the first to join the group. I would be the director of the CT Department and would have complete control over the scanning protocols and techs. My starting salary was to be twice as much as I was currently receiving.

At the end of the evening I told Gabe I would take the job. I would move to Michigan as soon as I obtained a Michigan medical license.

I was granted my license one month later. I drove through a winter storm to arrive in Wilno on February 20, 1987.

February twenty-fourth was my first day of work. Gabe gathered the technical staff in the angiography suite and said, "I want to introduce Dr. Duncan. He is the first radiologist to join our new group. Dr. Duncan is fellowship-trained in CT and interventional radiology. He is going to be a valuable asset to our department.

"There is one other issue to discuss. I will say this only once. I know who the troublemakers are in this room. Today I am wiping the slate clean. We are starting over. This is Day One in our department. From this moment forward there will be no dissension here. You will not give Dr. Duncan or me one scintilla of grief. If Dr. Duncan tells you to repeat a chest X-ray, you will provide him with one. If he wants a syringe, you will bring him one. If he wants extra views of the kidneys on a pyelogram, you will perform extra views. I want Dr. Duncan to be completely satisfied with your work."

It was just Gabe and I running the entire department the first month. We each did an enormous amount of work every day and we alternated taking call every other night. We hung on for dear life until reinforcements arrived. When Mike Morris and Bob Percy arrived, our lives settled into a manageable routine. A few years later, Phil Carlson joined the group.

# *Chapter* 16

With Gabe's departure, we had to choose a new chairman. I was not a suitable candidate. I had already alienated George Gravy and Martin Gesso. In addition, the guys knew I refused to involve myself in the small details of running the department, such as finances and work schedules. I relied on others to get their hands dirty.

Phil had a poor relationship with many of the techs. He frequently called them idiots and boneheads. There was certain to be a thick portfolio of complaints against Phil sitting in the administrative office.

Mike was too nice to be chairman. He didn't like confrontations. He didn't stand up to authority. His desire to please everyone could have been suicidal in those circumstances.

It was by default, therefore, that we chose Bob to be chairman. The problem with Bob was his enormous ego. He generally cared only about himself. Bob was a weightlifter and vain about his muscular physique. He took extraordinary measures to assert his virility and masculinity.

From the very beginning, we were not sure whose side Bob was on. He was not transparent about his dealings with administration. I was sure that Gravy and Gesso were flattering Bob by telling him how easy he was to work with, how willing he was to cooperate with them, in contrast with the rest of the radiologists. They were going to try to manipulate Bob by inflating his ego.

In May we were given a glimpse of the kind of department Bob wanted to create. Dr. Sam Charney, a hospital-employed general practitioner and general troublemaker, had come into Phil's office one morning at seven to complain about a report. None of the rads were in the department. Charney went to the front desk to ask our receptionist where the fuck the radiologists were. As always, he reeked of marijuana. Everyone in the hospital knew he used drugs. This was not a reportable offense, as he was a referring physician. Therefore he could expect immunity for pretty much anything short of mass murder.

Our receptionist told Charney that the radiologists started work at seven thirty and asked if he would like to leave a message. Charney explained that he did not want to leave a fucking message. Then he reported our dereliction of duty to administration. Thus it was that in May we were in Bob's office to deal with this latest crisis. Bob informed us that Martin Gesso had demanded that we start work at seven.

I exploded. "Why not six? Better yet, why don't we stay here twenty-four hours a day in case Charney comes in at midnight to complain about something? Our contract only requires that we start at eight. Charney has no right to decide when we come to work in the morning."

"Guys, my morning schedule is set in stone," Mike added. "I need to drop off my kids at school at exactly seven twenty. We are already here ten hours a day. One of us is on call twenty-four hours a day."

Bob expressed his concern that Gesso would not be pleased if we failed to comply with his ultimatum.

I spoke up. "Bob, I don't give a rat's ass if Gesso is not pleased. Our contract says we start work at eight. We can't start changing everything because some stoned-out troublemaker comes into our department and starts bitching about us. We need to have at least some control over our own department. I promise I will not come to work earlier."

The ball was in Bob's court. He was grinding his jaw and flexing his considerable biceps.

"Tim, I will have no power to pursue my agenda if I piss Gesso off. Let's just do what they want for a month. After that they will forget about the whole thing."

"Maybe they will forget about it," I said, "but we would be setting a precedent that we always cave in to their demands. They will think we are weak, and they will use that against us the next time our contract needs to be renewed."

"Speaking of our contract, Tim, it is coming up for renewal at the end of this year," Bob reminded.

Gabe said, "All the more reason to show them now that we are not going to join lockstep with every one of their idiotic demands. I believe the majority opinion here is that we are not coming to work earlier. There is no need to discuss it further. We are not going to change our starting time."

*Chapter* 17

June 21, 1998

The annual residents' and interns' graduation was held at the Rainbow Valley Country Club. Approximately thirty individuals would receive diplomas this year. Dinner would be served, speeches would be given, and diplomas would be distributed. Gabe and I sat with Fred and Karen Quimby. Joanie was home with the flu.

The attending physicians mingled and tried to ameliorate some of the bad blood created by our daily interactions. We pretended that, despite our hatred and distrust of each other, we still liked each other. We discussed such vital topics as whether our ties were really made in Italy, whether we had played golf this year, and whether our cars performed well in winter weather.

I congratulated as many of the graduates as possible for their achievement. My unspoken fear was probably similar to what people must feel when they bring children into the world during times of plague and famine.

The formal ceremony began as we finished our desserts. Normally the diplomas were handed out by the director of medical education, but a replacement had not yet been found for Jim Rowley following his forced resignation over the porcelain rhinoceros affair. George Gravy would be handing out the diplomas this year. Many of the physicians, including me, were offended at having a nonmedical person perform this function. I did not applaud when Gravy took the podium and began his speech.

"It is widely known that the practice of medicine is undergoing rapid and dramatic changes. In the case of Wilno General Hospital, we know that providers must be team players. They must be willing to work harder for less money, and to provide better service for the customer. Those providers who do not embrace this philosophy will not survive. The days of private practice are over. The providers of the future will be employed by the hospital or a health maintenance organization, also known as an HMO."

Or maybe it stands for "Handing Medicine Over," I thought.

George Gravy continued, "The future provider will wear a white coat displaying the hospital logo and will practice health care based on algorithms, which will be provided by the hospital administration. In the interest of cost containment, providers will not discuss treatment options with the customers. This policy has been forced on all of us because the current providers have been unable to control costs.

"The alarming increase in the cost of health care has been caused by medical technology. CT scans are expensive and unnecessary in most cases. Mammograms have been ordered in women who are only forty years old."

"Therefore, as I hand out each diploma, I will give each future provider a can of Campbell's chicken soup. It is widely known that chicken soup has considerable curative properties. If our customers ate more chicken soup, they would be healthier and would not need the expensive care required with more advanced diseases."

This was too much to bear. George Gravy was embarrassing himself and making a mockery of the hospital. Somebody had to do something.

Gabe, bless his heart, stood and addressed George Gravy.

"Mr. Gravy, chicken soup may be fine to treat the common cold, but do you seriously believe that chicken soup can prevent or treat breast cancer? Should we start giving chicken soup to a patient in the ER with a ruptured spleen?"

There was a stunned silence in the auditorium. I loved Gabe Watson. I wanted to hoist him on our shoulders and sing "For He's a Jolly Good Fellow." He had exposed George Gravy as the blockhead he really was.

Gravy was outraged. "Dr. Watson, you are being disruptive. Take your seat or I will call security."

As the director of the CT department, I couldn't allow myself to be neutral. I rose to stand next to Gabe and whispered, "Gabe, let's walk out. I can't stand to listen to any more of this garbage, and I don't want them to throw you out."

Gabe and I walked out of the building. Enough was enough. It was bad enough we had to endure these insufferable fools at work every day, but now they were trying to indoctrinate a whole new generation of physicians with their idiotic ideas. What was next? Leeches? Bloodletting?

*Chapter* **18**

The file clerk in the radiology department claimed that Phil had shoved her, causing bruising of her left buttock. It was June 25, and we were having yet another emergency meeting. Ben Gladstone, the department manager, was explaining the situation.

"Those assholes in administration have been telling the staff to make up negative stuff about you guys. We all know you didn't shove the file clerk, Phil. I'll pull her into my office this afternoon and see if I can resolve the situation. Don't worry, we will sort it out. I just wanted to alert you guys about what you are up against."

I tried to console Phil. He was worried. I would have been worried too. I told him the situation would be resolved. Ben was on our side. He would take care of things.

The next day the file clerk announced that she was married to Jesus Christ. It turned out she had schizophrenia and had stopped taking her medications. She was placed in a psychiatric hospital for evaluation.

Our administration told us that, in the interests of cost containment, they would not be hiring a new file clerk.

# Chapter 19

## July 1998

Summer was in full bloom and the weather was glorious. Joanie and I had been riding our bicycles around the neighborhood. Jasper and Cala were prowling around the backyard, eating grass and vomiting. Jasper ensnared a vole, defined by the Oxford English Dictionary as "a small, mouse-like rodent with a rounded muzzle" (I had to look it up). Jasper's pride in presenting his trophy to us was touching, and we lavished him with praise.

At WGH the general practitioners had launched a summer offensive against the specialists, with the full support of administration. The crisis of the hour revolved around the issue of electronic medical records (EMR). The providers were required to install EMR software into their office computer systems or they would face reductions in their future reimbursements. They informed the specialists that we should pool our financial resources to pay for their EMR software if we expected to receive any patient referrals in the future. I believe this is referred to as "extortion" in the legal community.

EMR represented a transition from the use of paper charts to the electronic collection and storage of patient information. It allowed communication with other providers who were connected to the system. It provided information about the drugs a physician was ordering, and performed a lot of other useful functions.

The major obstacle to offices wishing to install the system was cost. The system could cost upward of $15,000. I understood that the physicians were reluctant to spend their own money to install the systems, but what they were asking the specialists to do was illegal. There were anti-kickback regulations which prohibited specialists from giving money to their referring doctors.

An emergency meeting of the specialists was called one evening in the hospital auditorium. I was starting to feel like I was spending my whole life in emergency meetings. However, this one had a unique dimension. Trying to corral an assortment of specialists into making a collective decision has been aptly compared to trying to herd cats. The interests of a surgeon do not intersect with the interests of a pathologist.

One specialist pointed out that no one in the city was going to yield to such an outrageous demand, so the referring doctors would have to continue to send us their patients. Another said that he would have to install the EMR system in his own office, and he couldn't afford to pay for both his system and someone else's. A general surgeon pointed out that he was paying sixty thousand dollars a year for his malpractice insurance. Medicare was paying him three hundred dollars for a hernia repair and forty dollars for an office visit. He was in no position to contribute money.

We all agreed that the demand by the referring physicians was unreasonable, and that all of us would refuse to pay for their systems. I knew that this proclamation was disingenuous, though. Some of these guys would go running to pay for the software. This was their chance to grow their share of the pie. They would be able to undercut their competition. They would show the referring physicians that they understood who buttered their bread.

$Chapter$ **20**

My role in the department revolved around our $1.4 million third-generation CT scanner. I was fortunate to have been named director of the CT department, since it was my favorite modality. The amount of useful information that was obtained was staggering.

One of the more interesting aspects of CT scanning is that, in addition to addressing the primary indication of the study— i.e., does an enlarged liver contain a tumor—the scan sometimes detects unexpected findings which may be more important than the answer to the primary question.

The "incidental finding" is a mixed blessing. Most have no clinical significance, and referring physicians were annoyed when we found a tiny lung nodule in a lung base when all they cared about was the evaluation of the liver. But we were required to report every finding on a study. Due to the remarkable resolution of our studies, we were able to detect lung nodules the size of a piece of rice. We routinely reported tiny lung nodules, benign adenomas in the adrenal glands, benign vascular lesions in the liver, and thyroid nodules. The way the radiologist reports these findings is critical. While it is remotely possible that a tiny solitary lung nodule represents a metastatic cancer, the chances are so remote that I usually didn't even mention the possibility. Merely putting the word "cancer" in the conclusion of the report has major psychological and medical implications. I generally just said "incidental finding of a small lung nodule, most consistent with a benign granuloma." Some radiologists would tell me I was crazy to not even mention the possibility of cancer. Others would agree with my reporting method.

Many of our referring physicians would have preferred us not to detect incidental findings. I did not blame them. We sometimes created needless anxiety, and additional follow-up studies might be required. However, from my perspective, incidental findings could sometimes provide huge benefits for the patient.

The best example of this involved one of our ER physicians. He was fifty-five years old and had experienced the classic signs and symptoms of diverticulitis, a very common condition. We were asked to perform an abdominal CT to evaluate the extent of his disease. The study demonstrated a relatively mild case of inflammation of the descending colon, which should respond to a course of antibiotic therapy.

Of far greater importance was the fact that there was a small solid mass in the periphery of his left kidney. Based on the mass's characteristics, I suspected it represented a malignancy. It was small, about the size of an olive, and peripheral, so there would be no clinical signs of renal cancer, such as blood in his urine. This was a serendipitous finding.

The referring physician took my report and ordered a consult with one of our urologists.

I also told the patient about my finding. I knew from experience that this was the type of finding that could easily fall through the cracks. The urologist was "old school." He did not trust CT scans and did not like having to rely on the radiology report. He trusted the urinalysis. If the patient did not have blood in his urine, then he didn't have a renal cancer.

I informed the urologist that it would be easy to perform a CT-guided fine-needle aspiration biopsy (FNAB) of the mass. He wanted to do a renal angiogram instead. I felt this was a mistake, but there was no point in arguing with him. He was a very stubborn individual and was not going to listen to me, a mere radiologist.

The angiogram was performed at an outside hospital. The surgeon wanted to show us that he didn't trust anyone in our department to perform the study. The angiogram was reported to be normal. The surgeon told me that this proved my diagnosis was wrong. I told the surgeon that my diagnosis was not wrong. I told the patient that my diagnosis was not wrong.

I got Gabe involved, as he was the best angiographer in our department. I asked him to review the images from the outside hospital. After he reviewed the study, he called the urologist and me into his office.

"The angiogram was reported as normal," Gabe said. "However, I did some magnification of the images, and there is a tiny feeder vessel to the mass, and a small vascular blush. These findings are barely visible, but they are real findings."

I looked at the magnifications and agreed with Gabe. I was impressed. Gabe was really good when it came to angiography. The surgeon didn't bother to look at the magnification views.

"I could do an FNAB of the mass," I offered.

The surgeon finally agreed to the biopsy. It came back positive for cancer. The surgeon performed a simple wedge resection of the cancer, and the patient retained full function of his left kidney.

This case brought me a lot of personal satisfaction. My persistence had paid off. The cancer could have killed the patient in five years.

Even after this, the surgeon continued to question my reports. He probably thought this case proved nothing. I had never blown a diagnosis on his patients, but he didn't care. I didn't care that he didn't care. The patient, the ER physician, had thanked me for doing such a good job. That was reward enough.

$$Chapter\ 21$$

The biggest headache of being in charge of the CT department was patient scheduling. Doctors became hysterical when they had to wait a day for an inpatient scan. They were being closely monitored to insure that they kicked their patients out of the hospital as quickly as possible. I spent too much time on the telephone, explaining that we really, truly did not have any open slots that day for studies that were not emergencies. Some would say, "Well fine, I will order it as an emergency study. It is an economic emergency." I would reply that I did not appreciate intellectual dishonesty, but that if they ordered the study as an emergency, I would have to remove one of their other patients from the day's schedule. This usually resolved the problem, although I had the phone slammed down on me more than once.

As it was, we were cranking out our studies at the rate of one patient every twelve minutes, all day, every day, Monday through Friday. In spite of our hectic schedule, we were barely keeping up with demand. The techs did an outstanding job, as I frequently told them. I did everything I could to encourage and support them. They were scanning fifty patients a day. I had a nice lunch brought in for them once a week.

*Chapter* **22**

It was during the summer of 1998 that Martin Gesso delivered the ultimatum that would turn me from being a fairly nice person into a vicious attack dog. Administration had been tormenting our department the entire year and told us a day of reckoning was coming. They couldn't stand the fact that we were making a lot of money, and they said openly that they wanted to get rid of us. They were acting like idiots. We were making more money for the hospital than any other department. They should have been giving us their full support. Instead they thought we should be underpaid hospital employees, or else we should be eliminated. If they got their hands on the interpretation fees, they could increase the hospital revenues. They could also justify giving themselves large bonuses at the end of the year.

The pretense for the ultimatum was a meeting Gesso set up with us to ask if we wanted to provide coverage for a small upstate outpatient clinic that WGH wanted to acquire. We explained that we could not provide coverage, as our resources were already stretched to the limit. Gesso seemed to accept our explanation. I just wanted the meeting to end so I could get back to work. However, Gesso had one more item he wished to discuss with us. He explained that the hospital needed to generate more revenue, and that he expected us to agree to become employees of the hospital at our contract renewal at the end of the year. He told us what our salary would be. It was less than half of what we were currently earning.

"The radiologists need to take a pay cut for the good of the hospital," Gesso explained.

"Mr. Gesso," I said, "what kind of pay cut are you and the vice presidents going to take for the good of the hospital? Let's talk about that for a while. Then let's talk about the $9 million a year our department already generates for the hospital. You keep talking about how we are all on the same team, but it seems your concept of being a team only runs in one direction."

"Dr. Duncan, it is necessary for administration to be paid competitively so we can attract top talent to the hospital."

"Wouldn't the same argument apply to the radiologists?" I asked. "How are you going to have talented radiologists if you underpay them? Or maybe you don't care about the quality of the radiologists. Maybe you just want the cheapest guys you can find."

"Dr. Duncan, it is nonnegotiable that you will become employees. The salary we are offering is more than fair. You are currently making more than the vice presidents. No physician should make more money than the vice presidents."

"If we make more money than the vice presidents, it is because, unlike them, we actually contribute something to the hospital. Becoming a hospital employee is nonnegotiable with me. I won't do it. If you press this issue and we all resign, it will take you years to reestablish the kind of revenue we are currently generating. It may never happen. After I tell every radiologist in the country how you treat your radiologists, you will be lucky to find anyone willing to work at this hospital."

I walked out of the conference room and returned to my office. Gesso was pathetic. He hadn't heard a word I said. In his mind it would be easy to replace us. He was about to make a huge mistake, but he wouldn't listen to common sense because, after all, he was part of the almighty administration.

# Chapter 23

July 1998

I was sitting in the kitchen one Sunday afternoon, putting the finishing touches on a lecture I was going to give to the medical staff, when the idea came to me. It came in a rudimentary form, but I couldn't get it out of my mind. I wandered around in the backyard for a while as I thought. I recalled the lunchroom bitching sessions with the private practice physicians. One of them had said administration told the ER physicians to send only the patients with no insurance to them for follow-up care. Another said his group had missed out on a big contract with an insurance company because Gesso had refused to cosign the contract. They were all tired of the economic warfare.

My idea started to take shape. What would happen, I wondered, if the private practice physicians organized a coalition to fight back against administration? Doubts crept into my mind. If we just formed a group of physicians, it would turn into a social club. We would have an organization, but we would still just be bitching among ourselves. That wouldn't accomplish anything.

Finally the answer came to me. We could form a group that included influential members of the community. We could take our agenda outside the hospital. Surely the local community would be interested in learning more about health care issues. If we could present ourselves properly, maybe we could put pressure on the hospital to stop harassing us.

I came up with a name for the organization. We would call ourselves the Citizen's Health Alliance with Medical Professionals, CHAMP for short. I got out a pen and paper and outlined my plan. Then I decided to put my plan into action. At the end of the evening, Joanie told me I had a devilish grin on my face.

I had to find out if my idea was viable. The next day at work I ran the idea past a few of the private practice physicians. They thought it was a great idea. I told them to let anyone who might be interested know that I was holding a meeting at my house the following Saturday evening.

Eighteen private practice physicians converged on our house on Saturday evening. The rads were there too. I asked Gabe to introduce me, though it was a formality.

Gabe said, "As you know, Tim comes up with some pretty wacky ideas at times, but this is something I think we all want to hear about. So I immediately yield the floor to him."

I began by evoking the opening sentence of Karl Marx's *Communist Manifesto*. I had always wanted to do this at least once in my life. "Colleagues, the specter of managed care is sweeping across the country. Private practice is under assault. The administration is hostile. We should organize ourselves to resist administration. I want to take our message to the community.

I have a plan of action, but before I tell you my plan, are there are any questions?"

Kurt Jonas, a general surgeon and a good friend of mine, asked, "Tim, whom are you going allow to be in CHAMP? "

"There is only one requirement: you cannot be a supporter of the current administration. Does anyone here support these morons? If so, we certainly should hear your opinion."

No one supported the current administration.

Gabe made a motion to form CHAMP as a formal organization. The motion was approved unanimously. We were five minutes into the meeting. In the sixth minute I was elected president. By the seventh minute I was explaining my plan.

"Here is part one. I am going to have some small, tasteful stickers printed up which will say, 'Welcome to my private practice.' I ask that you place one of the stickers on the window by your front desk.

"Here is part two. I want to expose the local community to CHAMP. I was able to get Christ Church to donate the use of their auditorium on Saturday night, two weeks from today. I want six of you to give a ten-minute talk on a health care topic related to your specialty. I am going to say nice things about all of you guys in my opening remarks. Kurt, I want you to go first and talk about gastroesophageal reflux disease.

"Here is part three. I want you all to invite everyone you can think of to attend our event. I especially want to attract influential members of the community. I am going to notify the local newspaper about the event.

"Here is part four. This part is important. I want you to spread the word about the event. I want people at the hospital to know about it. In particular I want George Gravy to hear about it."

*Chapter* **24**

The Christ Church auditorium held about two hundred people. It was about half full when I took the podium. George Gravy was seated in the third row.

I began my opening remarks. "I want to thank you all for coming tonight. My name is Timothy Duncan. I am a private practice radiologist at Wilno General Hospital. One of the goals of the CHAMP organization is to promote community health through education. We have some outstanding private practice physicians lined up tonight to give you an overview of community health issues. I hope you will find their talks to be helpful and informative.

"The other mission of CHAMP is to alert the community to the danger that, without your support, the private practice physician may soon be extinct. There are forces in the current practice environment that make it increasingly difficult for private practices to survive.

"I have a case to make for private practice physicians. There are no barriers to having an open discussion about your health care options. They are not functioning under any gag orders which would prevent them from discussing alternative treatment plans."

George Gravy rose from his seat and started to gather his things as if to leave. He and I stared at each other for a full thirty seconds. He coughed once and then sat down.

"I would like to introduce our first speaker, Dr. Kurt Jonas. He is an expert in all areas of general surgery, but especially with gastrointestinal procedures. He is going to talk about the surgical treatment of gastroesophageal reflux disease."

I hoped the irony was not lost on Gravy. One of my goals tonight was to induce a case of heartburn in his gullet.

Kurt gave an excellent presentation. The remaining lectures also went well. At the end of the lectures I again thanked the audience and told them we would have another event in the fall.

George Gravy approached me and said he did not appreciate my remarks about managed care. He also did not think I should be using the term "gag orders."

"Mr. Gravy, I never used the term 'managed care,'" I pointed out. "Regarding the gag order, I was merely referring to your remarks at the graduation ceremony. You said the providers of the future should not discuss treatment options with patients. By the way, thank you for coming tonight. Please tell administration we are going to have more of these events."

"Are you ever going to ask one of the hospital-employed physicians to give a lecture?"

"Mr. Gravy, if I were you, I wouldn't hold my breath."

I was next approached by a well-dressed, middle-aged woman who identified herself as the president of the local Business Leaders Association.

"Dr. Duncan, every member of the community should be attending these lectures. Here is my business card. Please inform me when you set a date for your next event. I want to run an editorial letter in the newspaper and urge everyone to attend. By the way, how can the public know which physicians are in private practice?"

"You just need to call their offices and ask," I replied. "Many are not yet members of CHAMP. The CHAMP members will have a sticker in their offices that will say, 'Welcome to my private practice.'"

The last person to approach me was a newspaper reporter. He wanted to schedule an interview with me for the following week.

The day after the event, Ben Gladstone came into my office. As department manager, he had been sent to deliver a message.

"Tim, you have really stirred up a hornet's nest. Those assholes in administration said to tell you they don't want any more remarks about gag orders."

"So they want to issue a gag order about talking about gag orders?"

"That's an interesting way to put it. Listen, I think what you guys are doing is great. Let them stew in their juices. Do you have a reply you want me to give them?"

"Sure, Ben. You can ask them if they want to give me a presentation as to why I am not entitled to free speech. We can meet in my office. Tell them to keep it brief, as I have patient responsibilities. You can also tell them to watch for my interview in the newspaper about CHAMP. It should be coming out next week."

I had never seen Ben laugh so hard. "Tim, you know I am not going to tell them that."

"No, Ben, probably not," I said.

# Chapter 25

Eighteen new people joined CHAMP in August, bringing our total membership to thirty-seven, including me.

Martin Gesso unwittingly provided us with seventeen new members. At a meeting with the entire nursing staff, he told them he was going to reduce their wages by one dollar an hour, and that some of them would be laid off. The nurses were outraged. One of the head nurses confronted Gesso. She pointed out that he was making close to a million dollars a year and was driving an $80,000 car. She said it should be him taking a pay cut. Gesso tried to defend himself by claiming that he had no control over his salary and that it was determined by the board of directors. The nurses were not appeased. They threatened a class action lawsuit.

They would go to the media. Their husbands might beat him up. It was easy to recruit seventeen of them to join CHAMP.

We gained another member under bizarre circumstances. This woman was one of the legal advisers to the hospital. She had brought some hospital Medicare violations to the attention of Mr. Gesso and been promptly fired. Her husband was a federal prosecutor with connections in Washington, DC. They were planning to file a whistleblower action against the hospital. She was happy to join our group.

I wrote a letter to the board of directors on behalf of CHAMP, spelling out our various grievances. I pointed out that Gesso and his minions had alienated the entire nursing staff and most of the private practice physicians, and had exposed the hospital to charges of Medicare fraud. I demanded that the entire administration be fired.

I realized how audacious my actions were, but I was doing nothing illegal or improper. I wanted to see how far I could go in annoying these guys. If they were smart, they would just ignore me. They could let the clock run out on our contract and I would be gone in four months. But I wanted them to know how miserable those four months were going to be for them.

$Chapter$ **26**

## September 1, 1998

It was my forty-seventh birthday. As I sat in my office, I knew that events were coming to a head.

The previous evening I had received a phone call from Daniel Collins at the Sykes Recruiting Agency. Years ago I had sent them my c.v. to keep in their files. I had no interest in changing jobs at that time, but it never hurt to do a little snooping. Daniel had told me that there was an exciting job opportunity in my part of the state. I asked him for the name of the hospital that was searching for a radiologist.

"Dr. Duncan, I have it right here," Daniel said. "It is Wilno General Hospital."

"When do they want the person to start work?"

"They are in a bit of a rush. They need someone to start on October first of this year."

"Did they say why they needed a new radiologist so soon?" I asked.

"They said they couldn't work with the present group. They said the present group is too disruptive. They are going to cancel their contract this week."

"Daniel, I like you, so don't think that I am angry at you, but if you double-check my c.v. you will find that I am part of the group currently working at Wilno General. I'm sure you just made an honest mistake."

There was a pause. "Oh my God," Daniel said. "Oh my God. Dr. Duncan, I am so sorry about the mistake."

"Daniel, don't worry about it. Anyone can make a mistake. In fact, I am glad you called. I think we should just keep this conversation to ourselves. Call me again if you have another job opportunity."

I immediately called the other rads to tell them about the conversation.

# Chapter 27

So there I was on my birthday, having lunch with Seth Davis. He had just finished telling me a joke that was making the rounds. I laughed and said, "Seth, I have an even better joke. All of the radiologists are going to be replaced at the end of the month, if not sooner."

"Tim, are you serious?"

"As a bowel obtruction."

"Are you sure? Are you sure the administration isn't going to renew your contract?"

"Gesso told us we would have to become hospital employees or else he would get rid of us. We are not going to stay here and make half of what we could make somewhere else."

"Tim, those assholes have been telling the anesthesiologists that we are going to become employees too. It's a joke, because we bought all of our equipment from the hospital before Browning left."

"That was a smart move, Seth. Unfortunately, the rads didn't have a few million dollars sitting around to buy our equipment."

Seth shook his head. "This is going to cause a shit storm. I've got to tell Peter about this. He will be furious. He thinks you guys are the best radiology group in the whole city."

Cardiologist Peter Murphy was in my office an hour later. "Seth told me you guys are going to be replaced at the end of the month."

"If not sooner, Peter."

"But you guys are the best we have ever had."

"Tell that to administration," I muttered.

"I just came from administration. Those idiots have locked themselves in their offices. They refused to come out to talk with me."

"Did you try a stun grenade?"

"Shit," Peter said. "Shit, shit, shit."

Ten minutes after Peter left my office, five guys in polyester suits charged into the department and gave each of us a certified letter that our contract had been cancelled. We were going to be replaced at the end of the month. After the stormtroopers shoved the letters in our faces, they went downstairs and stuffed identical letters into the mailboxes of the entire medical staff. The letters did not specify the reasons our contract had been cancelled. We were simply accused of being disruptive and unprofessional.

We all gathered in Gabe's office. I had a very specific plan in mind. I wanted to file a lawsuit on the grounds of harassment and illegal contract cancellation. The rest of the group didn't know what they wanted to do.

We had a meeting with our attorney. The group was deeply divided. I was adamant that the hospital could not prove its allegations. Our lawyer agreed with me but said that a lawsuit would involve considerable time and expense. The rest of the group just wanted to receive compensation for the time remaining on our contract. We all wanted to leave. The situation was a nightmare. We were exhausted.

Our lawyer suggested a compromise. We would propose that the hospital compensate us for the time left on our contract and provide positive letters of reference in the future. In return we would refrain from filing a lawsuit. The group voted to accept his plan.

The hospital agreed to our proposal. At the end of the month we simply walked away from the hospital, never to return.

A couple of weeks after we left our jobs, Peter Murphy called me at home one evening to update me on developments.

"Tim, as of now we have no radiology department. They can't even find temporary replacements for you guys. We are sending all our work to other hospitals. If things stay this way, the hospital will be bankrupt within six months."

"And what will happen if the hospital goes bankrupt?"

"If we are lucky, we will be bought out by a large hospital chain."

"Does administration have anything to say for itself?" I asked.

"We haven't seen any of them for the past two weeks. The whole bunch of them have locked themselves in their offices. These sons of bitches have ruined the hospital. I wouldn't be surprised if they fled the country."

"There is always extradition."

"The hospital is never going to be the same. I don't think we are going to survive. I wish I could have done more for you guys."

"Peter, there was nothing more anyone could have done. Things would have turned out the same way. Listen, I have to go. Stay in touch."

# Epilogue

Joanie and I moved to Raleigh, North Carolina, at the end of 1998. We made the move for better weather, while still being relatively close to Joanie's family in Michigan. Joanie found a job at an outpatient oncology clinic. I worked at a couple of part-time jobs, but I mostly just chilled out and tried to figure out what to do with the rest of my life. We made a few trips to the Outer Banks. I did a couple of short-course triathlons and played golf.

Wilno General declared bankruptcy in the spring of 1999. The loss of revenues from the radiology department, and fines from Medicare violations, contributed to the bankruptcy. The hospital facility was sold to a national chain of nursing homes. The entire administration lost their jobs.

In 2003 we moved to Colorado Springs, Colorado, where Joanie's sister lives. We went hiking in the mountains nearly every weekend. I worked full time as a civilian contractor at the Air Force Academy Hospital. After five years I was laid off, along with a whole bunch of other contractors, as the result of a cost-saving move. It didn't bother me when this happened. We had saved enough money, and I retired at the age of fifty-seven.

We decided to move an hour north to Denver in 2008, where we remain to this day. We had so much fun for a couple of years that I rarely thought about my past life. I decided I might have a couple more triathlons left in my aging body, so I trained like a maniac and managed to complete a couple of events, although I was near the back of the pack.

I went through a brief phase where I thought about getting a post-graduate degree in philosophy and trying to teach at a university. But it would take three years to get a degree, and I would be too old by then to teach. Instead I hung out in book stores. I brought home books about the philosophers I had neglected during my undergraduate years.

I have no desire to return to the practice of medicine. It should be obvious that I am concerned about the future outlook for both physicians and patients. There will be a shortage of physicians as more of us begin to retire at a younger age. There was going to be a shortage anyway, but the developments of the past two decades will further aggravate that shortage.

I am glad for the ten good years I had at WGH. In those halcyon days I was able to devote all of my energy to interpreting medical images, teaching the residents, and maintaining my continuing medical education. My relatively large income allowed me to pay off my student loans, save for retirement, and live in a fairly nice house. But at the end of 1997 the dynamics at WGH completely changed. From that point on, even in my subsequent jobs, I was never able to really enjoy my work. Medicine had become a pure business. I always felt like an expendable cog in the health care machine. There was nothing fun or special about being a physician anymore.

I hope that nonmedical professionals, including political leaders and hospital administrators, will read my book and take my message seriously. Make no mistake. Physicians are under assault from every direction. We are leaving the professions in droves.

If President Obama and Congressional Democrats are sincere in their stated desire to reduce health care costs, they should address the issue of tort reform as soon as possible. Physicians are fully justified in calling for tort reform. The changes we ask for are not radical.

In legitimate cases of malpractice, patients should be fully compensated for their economic damages, with no limits on the amount of the award. Punative (noneconomic) damages should be capped at $300.000.00., except in extreme cases of malpractice. "Safe harbors" should be created for physicians who have practiced medicine within the standards of care, even when an individual patient has had a suboptimal outcome.

To conclude, the danger now exists that the profit motive has become the dominant dynamic in health care. Health care providers are judged by their ability to reduce corporate expences and increase corporate profits, rather than their clinical competence. This is not good for the autonomy and integrity that medicine requires. Indiividuals who have no knowledge of medicine have taken control. Of course these developments have made medicine a less attractive career choice. Current physicians are turning to early retirement. Talented young people may hesitate to pursue a creer in medicine. This may very well result in a significant physician shortage in the future.

# Bibliography

Halvorson, George C. "Health Care Will Not Reform Itself." 2009. CRC Press.

Lee, Thomas H., MD, Mongan,James J., MD. "Chaos and Organization in Health Care". 2009. The MIT Press.

Makary, Marty, MD., "Unaccountable". 2012. Bloomsbury Press.

Reid, T.R. "The Healing of America." 2010. Penguin Books.

Ruggieri, Paul A., MD. "Confessions of a Surgeon". 2012. Berkley Books.

Tate, Nick J. "ObamaCare Survival Guide". 2012. Humanix Books.

www.ingramcontent.com/pod-product-compliance
Lightning Source LLC
Chambersburg PA
CBHW022106170526
45157CB00004B/1498

9 781481 186759